Jolie Jones lives in the South East of England with her husband Mark, their four grown up(ish) sons, her mum and dad & their two dogs – what could possibly go wrong?!

Having spent the last 20+ years raising her children, she wanted to try something new... it turned out that this was also for them!

The idea for *Mwah My Wishes Are Here* was born over a decade ago, something special for those she loves.

In her spare time Jolie is either with family and friends or watching true crime documentaries.

JOLIE JONES

MWAH!
My Wishes
Are Here

AUSTIN MACAULEY PUBLISHERS™

LONDON • CAMBRIDGE • NEW YORK • SHARJAH

A CIP catalogue record for this title is available from the British Library.

ISBN 9781035849529 (Paperback)
ISBN 9781035849536 (Hardback)

www.austinmacauley.com

First Published 2024
Austin Macauley Publishers Ltd®
1 Canada Square
Canary Wharf
London
E14 5AA

This book is dedicated to the wonderful family I was born to be with, the family I made and the future families yet to be created.

My beautiful friends who make my world a better place.

'My Mark', Harry, Jack, Lawson & Cam – You are my everything – XXXXgX.

Introduction

Everyone's life is as individual as their fingerprint, with different characters, experiences, and storylines.

We collect memories and people that shape us, share laughter and our lives with those we love, and strive to be the best versions of ourselves.

Experiencing love means we are destined to experience loss; this book offers you a chance to leave something behind for those you love and who love you.

This is your blueprint that people can refer to, so that there are no tough decisions to be made, recollections are clearer, and your memory serves as a constant guide.

Grief can be paralysing, can incite anger and confusion, and can skew your thoughts.

Leave no room for ambiguity.

Help your people find their new normal while reminiscing about the old.

"I don't want my death to define you, I want my life to inspire you. I am writing mine for you, my loved ones, some of whom I haven't even met yet. Thank you for loving me. Xxxxgx." – Jolie Jones.

Daughter, sister, wife, mother, friend, colleague, stranger.

Contents

THE END...

I've answered these hard questions, so you don't have to...

You've got this...

"There is no real ending. It's just the place where you stop the story."
FRANK HERBERT

 "Time After Time" (Cyndi Lauper)

THIS IS ME...

Legal Name: ....

Birth Name: ....

Nickname: ....

Birth Date: ....

Star Sign: ....

Birth Weight: ....

Birth Place: ....

Birth Parents: ....

Life Parents: ....

Height: ....

Eye Colour: ....

Hair Colour: ....

Shoe Size: ....

Dominant Hand: ....

Religion/Faith:...

My Favourite Feature:...

Is there a Family Tree: ....

Next of Kin:..

If there is no hope, you need to let me go: ✓ ✗

Blood Type:...

Organ Donor: ✓ ✗

Allergies: ....

Important Health Information: ....

....

Regular Medication: ....

....

NHS/Medical Number:..

NI Number:..

Birth Certificate: ....

Passport Number:...

Driving Licence Number: ....

I have a will: ✓   ✗

Where: ....

....

My Important Documents can be found:..................................

....

Solicitor/Lawyer Details: ....

....

Insurance details:...

....

Funeral Plan: ....

Phone Company: ....

Phone Password:...

Social Media Sites Information:..

....

....

Other:...

....

....

....

---

*"The things that make me different are
the things that make me ME."*

A.A. MILNE

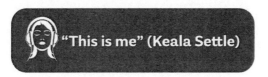

WHEN I PASS...

I would like to be dressed in: ....

....

I would like my hair to be: ....

....

I would like this make-up: ....

....

I would like to wear the following jewellery: ....

....

Other details: ....

....

....

....

I would like my coffin to be:...

....

In my coffin, I would like:...

....

On top of my coffin, I would like: ....

....

Viewings: If possible / No

Open coffin: If possible / No

I would like a Religious Service:....................................... ✓ ✗

    Where:...

I would like a Humanist Service: ✓ ✗

    Where:...

Other:...

I would like to be:

    Donated to Medical Science: ✓ ✗

Buried: ✓ ✗

Where:..

Who would you like to attend the burial? ....

....

....

I would like my headstone to be: ....

I would like my headstone to include:...

....

I would like to be cremated: ✓ ✗

Where:..

I would like my ashes to be:...

Kept: ✓ ✗

Scattered: ✓ ✗

Where: ....

....

Who to attend: ....

....

....

....

Other:...

....

....

....

I would like a plaque at:...

....

"Mine eyes are full of tears, my heart of grief."
WILLIAM SHAKESPEARE, HENRY VI

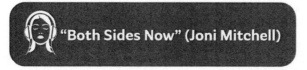

FOR MY SERVICE...

If possible, I would like to be driven from:..

....

Past: ....

Mode of transport:...

I would like my coffin to be in the venue before people arrive: ✓   ✗

I would like my coffin to arrive with my family after mourners
have arrived: ✓   ✗

Pallbearers to be: ....

....

Other:...

....

I would like the dress code to include: ....

....

....

I would like flowers: ✓ ✗

From: ....

I would like donations to the following charity: ....

....

I would like an order of service: ✓ ✗

Please can you include: ....

....

I would like the following music played:

Before: ....

....

During: ....

....

After: ....

....

Please do not play: ....

....

....

I would like the following readings: ....

....

....

....

Please do not read: ....

....

....

I would like photos to be taken: ✓ ✗

I would like the service/wake to be filmed: ✓ ✗

I would like a guestbook: ✓ ✗

I would like an obituary: ✓ ✗

 In: ....

Please include: ....

....

....

....

....

---

*"Grief cries and life shines on – and
hope paints a rainbow."*

TERRI GUILLEMETS

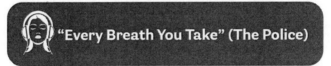 **"Every Breath You Take"** (The Police)

LET ME GUIDE YOU...

Information that can be included in Eulogy: ....

....

....

....

....

....

....

....

....

....

....

Significant milestones/information: ....

....

....

....

....

....

Significant people: ....

....

....

....

....

....

Academic/work achievements: ....

....

....

....

....

....

....

Family achievements: ....

....

....

....

....

....

....

Stories to be told:..

....

....

....

....

....

....

Please do not mention:..

....

....

....

....

....

....

Proudest moments: ....

....

....

....

....

Biggest life-changing decisions: ....

....

....

....

Greatest pieces of advice:...

....

....

....

....

I would like to thank:..

....

....

....

....

I hope I can be remembered this way:.................................

....

....

....

My hopes for you:..

....

....

....

If you see a: ....

....

.... think of me.

Find a place and make it ours: ....

....

....

....

---

*"Death is never a clean break – some
stardust always remains."*

TERRI GUILLEMETS

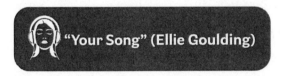

30

WAKE...

I would like the wake to be held at:..
....

I would like the event to be called:...
....

I would like a photo montage: ✓   ✗

 Including: ....
  ....

Speeches: ....
....
....

I would like a playlist: ✓   ✗

 Including: ....
  ....
  ....

I would like a guestbook: ✓ ✗

I would like the food served to include:..

....

....

I would like the drinks served to include:...

....

....

Any additional information: ....

....

....

---

*"Life may not be the party we hoped for, but
while we are here we should dance."*
AUTHOR UNKNOWN

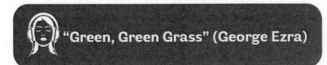 **"Green, Green Grass" (George Ezra)**

NEW NORMAL...

This is what I wish for you: ....

....

Daily: ....

....

....

....

Weekly: ....

....

....

....

Monthly: ....

....

....

....

Yearly:..

....

....

....

"Remember, hope is a good thing, maybe the
best of things and no good thing ever dies."

STEPHEN KING

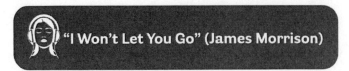 **"I Won't Let You Go" (James Morrison)**

MY ADVICE ON...

Work: ....

....

....

Life Hacks: ....

....

....

Regrets:...

....

....

Money:..

....

....

Moving House: ....

....

....

Birthdays: ....

....

....

Childbirth: ....

....

....

Parenthood: ....

....

....

Love: ....

....

....

Relationships: ....

....

....

Marriage: ....

....

....

Living with someone: ....

....

....

Family: ....

....

....

In-Laws: ....

....

....

Friends: ....

....

....

School: ....

....

....

Education: ....

....

....

Sex: ....

....

....

Dealing with loss: ....

....

....

Health: ....

....

....

Cosmetic Surgery: ....

....

....

Alcohol/Drugs: ....

....

....

Dealing with negative people/situations: ....

....

....

Siblings: ....

....

....

Loved ones moving on: ....

....

....

My partner moving on: ....

....

....

Feeling Lonely: ....

....

....

Other: ....

....

....

....

....

"Everything will be ok in the end. If it's not ok, it's not the end."

JOHN LENNON

 "I Hope You Dance" (Lee Ann Womack)

MIDDLE...

"A story should have a beginning, a middle and
an end, but not necessarily in that order."
JEAN-LUC GODARD

 "Young Hearts Run Free" (Candi Staton)

THESE ARE A FEW OF MY FAVOURITE THINGS...

Smell:..

Perfume/Aftershave:..

Colour:...

Animal:..

Haircut:...

Number: ....

Lottery Numbers:...

Name: ....

Noise:..

Day: ....

Month: ....

Star sign:...

Time:...

Decade:..

Word:...

Accent:..

Charity:...

Royal/President:...

Historical Figure:...

Historical Event:..

Law:...

Pet Name:...

Love Song:...

Party Song:..

Song:...

Singer: ....

Band: ....

DJ: ....

Radio Station: ....

Musician: ....

Artist: ....

Designer: ....

Style: ....

Gemstone: ....

Actor: ....

Programme: ....

Series: ....

Theatre Production: ....

Movie: ....

Scene in a Film:..

Magazine: ....

Newspaper: ....

Author:...

Book:...

Comedy: ....

Comedian:..

Presenter: ....

Dance:...

Night out: ....

Night In:...

Sleeping Position: ....

Board Game: ....

SPA Treatment:...

Car: ....

Method of Transport: ....

Household Chore: ....

Sport to Play: ....

Sport to Watch: ....

Athlete: ....

Form of Exercise: ....

Hobby: ....

Political Party: ....

Era: ....

Religion/Faith: ....

Weather: ....

Season: ....

View: ....

Beach: ....

Flower: ....

Walk: ....

Favourite Place: ....

Holiday Destination: ....

Country: ....

County/State: ....

Holiday Season: ....

Holiday Tradition: ....

Family Tradition: ....

Bar: ....

Restaurant: ....

Hotel: ....

Shop: ....

Flavour: ....

Food: ....

Meal of the Day: ....

Drink: ....

'Drink' Drink: ....

Takeaway: ....

Birthday: ....

Job: ....

Superpower: ....

Body Part: ....

Party Trick: ....

Daily Fix: ....

Skill: ....

Guilty Pleasure: ....

Joke: ....

Takeaway: ....

Superstition:..

Values:..

Qualities in a Person:...

Letter I have received: ....

Email I have received: ....

Gift I have been given:...

Gift I have given:...

Compliment: ....

Piece of Advice: ....

Quirks: ....

Quote: ....

Memories: ....

Other: ....

....

....

....

"It's not that I can't live without you,
it's just that I don't want to try."

ANON

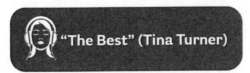 **"The Best" (Tina Turner)**

LEAST FAVOURITE...

Smell: ....

Perfume/Aftershave: ....

Colour: ....

Animal: ....

Haircut: ....

Number: ....

Name: ....

Noise: ....

Day: ....

Month: ....

Star Sign: ....

Time: ....

Decade:...

Word:..

Accent:...

Charity:..

Royal/President:..

Historical Figure:...

Historical Event:..

Law:..

Pet Name:...

Love Song:..

Party Song:...

Song:..

Singer:..

Band:..

DJ: ....

Radio Station: ....

Artist: ....

Musician: ....

Designer: ....

Style: ....

Gemstone: ....

Actor: ....

Programme: ....

Series: ....

Theatre Production: ....

Movie: ....

Scene in a Film: ....

Magazine: ....

Newspaper: ....

Author: ....

Book: ....

Comedy: ....

Comedian: ....

Presenter: ....

Dance: ....

Night Out: ....

Night In: ....

Sleeping Position: ....

Board Game: ....

Spa Treatment: ....

Car: ....

Method of Transport: ....

Household Chore: ....

Sport to Play: ....

Sport to Watch: ....

Athlete: ....

Form of Exercise: ....

Hobby: ....

Political Party: ....

Era: ....

Religion/Faith: ....

Weather: ....

Season: ....

View: ....

Beach: ....

Flower: ....

Walk: ....

Place: ....

Holiday Destination: ....

Country: ....

County/State: ....

Holiday Season: ....

Family Tradition: ....

Bar: ....

Restaurant: ....

Hotel: ....

Shop: ....

Flavour: ....

Food: ....

Meal of the Day: ....

Drink: ....

'Drink' Drink: ....

Takeaway: ....

Birthday: ....

Job: ....

Superpower: ....

Body Part: ....

Party Trick: ....

Skill: ....

Guilty Pleasure: ....

Joke: ....

Superstition: ....

Values: ....

Quality in a Person: ....

Letter I have received: ....

Email I have received: ....

Gift I have been given: ....

Gift I have given: ....

Compliment: ....

Piece of Advice: ....

Quirks: ....

Quotes: ....

Memory: ....

Other:..

> *"One man's trash is another man's treasure, what*
> *he doesn't appreciate, the next man will."*
>
> UNKNOWN

 "I Don't Like Mondays" (The Boomtown Rats)

I BELIEVE IN...

Aliens:	✓	✗	Abortion:	✓	✗
Other Worlds:	✓	✗	Euthanasia:	✓	✗
Forgiveness:	✓	✗	The Death Penalty:	✓	✗
Superstitions:	✓	✗	Taxes:	✓	✗
Apocalypse:	✓	✗	National Health Service:	✓	✗
Zombies:	✓	✗	Double Denim:	✓	✗
Fairy Tales:	✓	✗	War:	✓	✗
Luck:	✓	✗	Numerology:	✓	✗
The Monarchy:	✓	✗	Star Signs:	✓	✗
Democracy:	✓	✗	Religion:	✓	✗
Politics:	✓	✗	Faith:	✓	✗
In a Class System:	✓	✗	Life After Death:	✓	✗
Immigration:	✓	✗	Clairvoyants:	✓	✗
Animal Testing:	✓	✗	Ghosts:	✓	✗
Veganism:	✓	✗	Guardian Angels:	✓	✗

Hunting:	✓	✗	Use By Dates:	✓	✗
Education:	✓	✗	Immunisations:	✓	✗
Fate:	✓	✗	Competition:	✓	✗
Karma:	✓	✗	God:	✓	✗
Love At First Sight:	✓	✗	The Big Bang:	✓	✗
Mindfulness:	✓	✗	Time Travel:	✓	✗
Positive Mental Attitude:	✓	✗	Conspiracy Theories:	✓	✗
Organ Donation:	✓	✗	Attitude to Gratitude:	✓	✗
Cosmetic Surgery:	✓	✗	Regrets:	✓	✗
Marriage:	✓	✗	Attitude to Gratitude:	✓	✗
Manners:	✓	✗	Miracles:	✓	✗
Tipping:	✓	✗			

---

*"Never believe anything that requires you
to hate people who do not believe it."*

ROBERT BRAULT

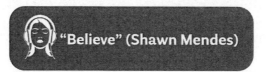

"Believe" (Shawn Mendes)

MY MAP...

Where I have lived, with whom and favourite memories: ....

....

....

....

....

....

....

....

*"My husband and I live with our four teenage
sons and my parents... it's like hosting a stag
party in an assisted living facility."*

JOLIE JONES

 "Where the Streets Have No Name" (U2)

NEVER HAVE I EVER...

Seen a Ghost:	✓	✗	Lied about My Age:	✓	✗
Been Arrested:	✓	✗	Won the Lottery:	✓	✗
Appeared on TV:	✓	✗	Been in a Helicopter:	✓	✗
Been on the Radio:	✓	✗	Had an Operation:	✓	✗
Been in the Paper:	✓	✗	Broken a Bone:	✓	✗
Won a Prize/Award:	✓	✗	Saved a Life:	✓	✗
Got a Tattoo:	✓	✗	Had Cosmetic Surgery:	✓	✗
Truanted:	✓	✗	Had an Emergency Wee:	✓	✗
Jumped out of a Plane:	✓	✗	Tried Drugs:	✓	✗
Stolen Anything:	✓	✗	Been Fired:	✓	✗
Seen a Clairvoyant:	✓	✗	Had a Near-Death Experience:	✓	✗
Got a Piercing:	✓	✗	Broken the Law:	✓	✗
Met a Member of the Royal Family/President:	✓	✗	Been Caught Speeding:	✓	✗
Met a Celebrity:	✓	✗	Cheated:	✓	✗

Been Cheated On: ✓ ✗

Sang Karaoke: ✓ ✗

Other: ✓ ✗

"Experience is the name everyone gives to their mistakes."
OSCAR WILDE

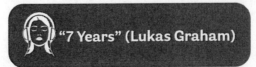 **"7 Years" (Lukas Graham)**

COULD HAVE, SHOULD HAVE, WOULD HAVE...

Opportunities, different choices and with hindsight: ....

....

....

....

....

I could have: ....

....

....

....

I should have: ....

....

....

....

....

I would have: ....

....

....

....

---

*"The only way you should look back is
with a big smile, or a wry one."*

JOLIE JONES

 "You can go your own way" (Fleetwood Mac)

CORPORATE CAGE...

Jobs, Career, Vocation, Volunteering: ....

....

....

Career Highlight: ....

....

....

Career Lowlight:...

....

....

"Your Brand is Your Name and Your Name is Your Brand."
DONALD KEITH BAKER

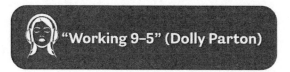 **"Working 9–5" (Dolly Parton)**

EDUCATION...

First Babysitter/Childminder/Nanny:..

First Nursery: ....

Infant School:...

Junior School:...

Playground Games: ....

Friends Were:...

Best Memories:..

Most embarrassing moment: ....

School Dinners were: ....

Packed Lunches were:...

Favourite subject: ....

Favourite Teacher: ....

What I wanted to be when I grew up:..

....

Senior School: ....

First Day: ....

Favourite Subject:..

Least Favourite Subject:...

Favourite Teacher & why: ....

Least favourite Teacher & why: ....

'Best' Life lesson learned: ....

Best Day:...

Worst Day:..

Most embarrassing moment: ....

Regrets: ....

Playground 'Rules':...

Popular Slang:...

School Dinners were: ....

Friendship Group:...

My advice to me would be:..

....

....

What I would change about the education system:.........................

....

....

College/Apprenticeship Scheme:...

University:...

Course: ....

Accommodation: ....

....

Staple Meal:..

Budget: ....

Typical night out: ....

Typical night in:...

Groups joined: ....

....

Advice I would give:..

....

....

Best Life Lesson learnt: ....

....

....

Other:..

....

....

"Life can only be understood backwards,
but it must be lived forwards."
SØREN KIERKEGAARD

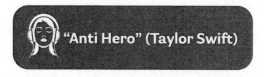

ROAD TRIP...

Where I have travelled, when, with whom and must do: ....

....

....

....

....

....

....

....

"Go forth. Act decent. Call your mother from time to time."
SIMCHA FISHER

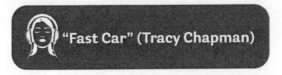 **"Fast Car"** (Tracy Chapman)

INFLUENCERS...

People who have influenced me: ....

....

....

....

....

Headlines that have changed my life: ....

....

....

....

....

Major events I have lived through:..

....

....

....

....

Strangers who have amazed me:...

....

....

....

....

Who deserves a cape:...

....

....

....

Who I have influenced: ....

....

....

....

....

....

If I had to live during a different Era, I would choose: ....

....

....

If I could have 6 people, excluding family & friends (alive or dead) for a
dinner party, this is who it would be and why?: ....

....

....

....

....

Kiss: ....

Marry: ....

Avoid: ....

Law you would amend/abolish: ....

....

....

Law you would amend/create: ....

....

....

Talent, I wish I had: ....

....

If I had 1 hour left, I would: ....

....

....

Bucket List:..

....

....

....

....

....

....

If I were a pigeon, I would poo on: ....

....

"If you would not ask someone for their advice, don't worry about their opinion."

UNKNOWN

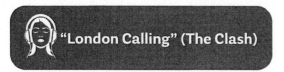 **"London Calling" (The Clash)**

I AM...

Honest:	...... /10	Creative:	...... /10
Loyal:	...... /10	Artistic:	...... /10
Faithful:	...... /10	Musical:	...... /10
Kind:	...... /10	A Good Singer:	...... /10
Funny:	...... /10	Dramatic:	...... /10
Attractive:	...... /10	Sentimental:	...... /10
Generous:	...... /10	A Hoarder:	...... /10
Maternal/Paternal:	...... /10	Adventurous:	...... /10
Comfortable in my own skin:	...... /10	A Traveller:	...... /10
A Homebody:	...... /10	Career Driven:	...... /10
A Party Animal:	...... /10	A DareDevil:	...... /10
DIY Legend:	...... /10	Academic:	...... /10
A Baker:	...... /10	Street Smart:	...... /10
A Good Cook:	...... /10	A Good Driver:	...... /10
		Clumsy:	...... /10

A Good Dancer:	...... /10	Good With Money:	...... /10
Stylish:	...... /10	Lucky:	...... /10
Trendy:	...... /10	Feisty:	...... /10
Lazy:	...... /10	Always Right:	...... /10
Caring:	...... /10	Forgiving:	...... /10
Stubborn:	...... /10	Naive:	...... /10
Impulsive:	...... /10	Shy:	...... /10
A Law Breaker:	...... /10	Houseproud:	...... /10
Positive:	...... /10	Outgoing:	...... /10
Competitive:	...... /10	Intelligent:	...... /10
A Leader:	...... /10	Family Orientated:	...... /10
A Follower:	...... /10	Driven By Money:	...... /10
Committed:	...... /10	Law Abiding:	...... /10
Loving:	...... /10	A Dog Lover:	...... /10
Comfortable with Public Displays of Affection (PDA):	...... /10	A Cat Lover:	...... /10
		Trustworthy:	...... /10
Opinionated:	...... /10		

A Goody Two Shoes:	...... /10	Spiritual:	...... /10
Naughty:	...... /10	A Glass Half Full person:	...... /10
A Movie Buff:	...... /10	Loud:	...... /10
Tardy:	...... /10	Polite:	...... /10
A Bookworm:	...... /10	Woke:	...... /10
A Water baby:	...... /10	Friendly:	...... /10
Moralistic:	...... /10	Confident:	...... /10
A Gym Bunny:	...... /10	Fashionable:	...... /10
Thoughtful:	...... /10	Streetwise:	...... /10
Romantic:	...... /10	Green Fingered:	...... /10
A Thrill seeker:	...... /10	An Early Bird:	...... /10
Old Fashioned:	...... /10	A Night Owl:	...... /10
A Hypochondriac:	...... /10	Compassionate:	...... /10
Flexible:	...... /10	Coordinated:	...... /10
Focused:	...... /10	Follically challenged:	...... /10
A workaholic:	...... /10	Jealous:	...... /10

Technical:	...... /10	A Chocoholic:	...... /10
Enthusiastic:	...... /10	Hyperactive:	...... /10
Well Mannered:	...... /10	Judgemental:	...... /10
Gossip:	...... /10	Thankful:	...... /10
Emotional:	...... /10		

Other:../10

..../10

..../10

..../10

..../10

..../10

"When you dance to your own rhythm,
life taps its toes to your beat."
TERRI GUILLEMETS

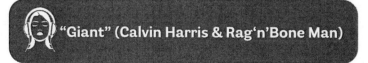

"Giant" (Calvin Harris & Rag'n'Bone Man)

DREAMS AND SCREAMS

Recurring/vivid dreams: ....

....

....

Recurring/vivid nightmares: ....

....

....

My phobias: ....

....

....

....

What makes me squeamish? ....

....

....

....

Biggest fear: ....

....

Scariest Moment: ....

....

Scariest film: ....

....

Regret: ....

....

....

....

*"Dreams are only thoughts you didn't have
time to think about during the day."*
AUTHOR UNKNOWN

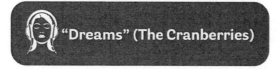 **"Dreams" (The Cranberries)**

SCARS, BREAKS AND LUCKY ESCAPES...

Scars I have acquired:..

....

....

Life changing diagnosis:...

....

Broken bones:...

....

....

Medical History:..

....

....

....

My body's weak area is: ....

....

Biggest challenges I have faced: ....

....

....

Lucky escapes: ....

....

....

Life is too short to/for:...

....

....

"Smooth seas do not make skilful sailors."
AFRICAN PROVERB

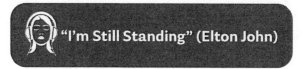 "I'm Still Standing" (Elton John)

FOOD FOR THOUGHT...

Family meals from childhood: ....

....

Family food traditions: ....

....

We Celebrate: ....

....

....

Food we celebrate with: ....

....

....

Family favourites: ....

....

....

Favourite Holiday Food:..

....

Food I cannot live without:...

....

....

Comfort Food:..

....

....

Strangest food you have eaten:..

....

Last meal:

    Starter:..

    ....

    Main:...

    ....

Sides: ....

....

Dessert: ....

....

Drink: ....

....

Other:...

....

....

....

....

"FHB – Family Hold Back."

 "Fairytale of New York" (The Pogues – Radio Version)

YOU CAN'T CHOOSE YOUR FAMILY...

Family Traditions: ....

....

....

Laughs, groans & what you wish to be continued: ....

....

....

Family Traits: ....

....

....

Quirks, attributes & lineage: ....

....

....

Family Folklore: ....

....

....

....

....

....

Stories and fables passed down: ....

....

....

....

....

"A family is a bunch of people who keep confusing
you with someone you were as a kid."
ROBERT BRAULT

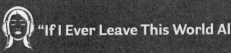 **"If I Ever Leave This World Alive" (Flogging Molly)**

YOU CAN CHOOSE
YOUR FRIENDS...

True friends, for a season or for a reason: ....

....

....

....

....

Where, how & when you met: ....

....

....

....

....

....

....

Favourite characteristics: ....

....

....

....

....

....

....

....

....

If you need to know..

....

....

....ask:

....

I bequeath: ....

....

....

....

....

....

*"You and I are more than friends, we're
like a really small gang."*

UNKNOWN

 "I'll Stand By You" (The Pretenders)

PHONE A FRIEND...

Who I would call if I needed...

A wingman:..

A Party Night:...

A Night In:...

Netflix & Chill: ....

Relationship Advice: ....

An Honest Opinion: ....

A Kick up the Backside: ....

Gift Ideas:..

A Belly Laugh:..

A Confidence Boost: ....

Work Advice: ....

Life Hacks: ....

Help Moving:..

Any DIY: ....

To Rant: ....

No Judgement: ....

Family Advice: ....

Children's Advice: ....

Life Advice: ....

Fashion Tips: ....

Someone to Just Listen: ....

A Calming Influence: ....

Practical Help: ....

To Remember/Reminisce: ....

An Adventure: ....

A Crossword Answer: ....

A Cuddle: ....

A Good Cry: ....

An Exercise Buddy: ....

Beautifying: ....

A Boozy Lunch: ....

A Cheeky Nando's: ....

An Alibi: ....

A Concert/Festival Friend: ....

To Borrow Something: ....

To Share A Secret: ....

A Good Debate: ....

A Casserole: ....

Movie recommendations: ....

If I needed Help In a Quiz: ....

The Truth: ....

To Go Out Of My Comfort Zone: ....

To Be Led Astray: ....

A Scapegoat: ....

An Excuse: ....

A Great Guest: ....

A Speech: ....

Word on the street: ....

Gossip: ....

A Fiver: ....

Other: ....

....

....

....

*"People are either your medicine or your
poison... choose medicine!"*

JOLIE JONES

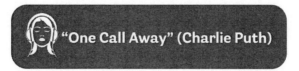
"One Call Away" (Charlie Puth)

RELATIONSHIPS AND SITUATIONSHIPS...

Best Chat-up line: ....

....

Worst Chat-up line: ....

....

Best Compliment: ....

....

Worst Insult: ....

....

Who should pay on the first date: ....

....

Best first date: ....

....

Worst first date: ....

....

Most romantic meal: ....

....

Most romantic holiday:...

....

Most romantic evening: ....

....

Most romantic gift: ....

....

Least romantic meal:..

....

Least romantic holiday:..

....

Least romantic evening: ....

....

Least romantic gift: ....

....

Been cheated on: ....

....

Cheated on: ....

....

Other: ....

....

....

"Never miss the forest for the trees."
JOHN HEYWOOD

 "We Go Together" (John Travolta & Olivia Newton-John)

SITUATIONSHIPS...

People you had a connection with, shared a moment with:.........................

....

....

Your usual 'type': ....

....

It's not me... it's you:...

....

What gives you the 'Ick'?...

....

---

*"In another life, I know we ended up together,
but in this one, I will just miss you."*

UNKNOWN

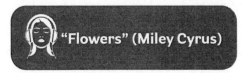 **"Flowers" (Miley Cyrus)**

RELATIONSHIPS...

Long-term relationships:...

....

....

First true love: ....

Stop-gaps: ....

....

....

The One:...

    The Proposal: ....

    The ring: ....

    Engagement Party: ✓   ✗

    How long was the engagement?...

    Wedding/Commitment Ceremony:..

....

Gift given to partner: ....

Gift received from partner: ....

Where: ....

When: ....

Time: ....

Any traditions: ....

....

....

Rings: ....

Photos/Film: ✓   ✗

Who gave you away: ....

Ceremony outfits: ....

....

Bridesmaids/Groomsmen:..

....

....

Gifts given to bridal parties: ....

Colour scheme: ....

Flowers: ....

How many guests: ....

Ceremony songs: ....

....

....

Readings: ....

....

....

Personal Vows: ....

....

....

....

Reception venue: ....

....

Wedding breakfast: ....

....

Speeches: ....

Guest Book: ✓ ✗

Entertainment: ....

Additional extras: ....

....

....

DJ/Band: ....

First dance: ....

Most vivid memory: ....

....

....

Funniest moment: ....

....

....

Most emotional moment: ....

....

....

What I may have done differently? ....

....

....

Wedding night was at:..

Favourite Gift received: ....

Other Details:...

....

....

Honeymoon: ....

"Love is an act of courage."

PAULO FREUD

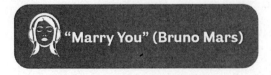

TAKE TWO...

The One: ....

The Proposal: ....

The ring: ....

Engagement Party: ✓ ✗

How long was the engagement? ....

Wedding/Commitment Ceremony: ....

....

Gift given to partner: ....

Gift received from partner: ....

Where: ....

When: ....

Time: ....

Any traditions: ....

....

....

Rings: ....

Photos/Film: ✓ ✗

Who gave you away: ....

Ceremony outfits: ....

....

Bridesmaids/Groomsmen:...

....

....

Gifts given to bridal parties: ....

Colour scheme:...

Flowers: ....

How many guests:..

Ceremony songs: ....

....

....

Readings: ....

....

....

Personal Vows: ....

....

....

....

Reception venue: ....

....

Wedding breakfast: ....

....

Speeches: ....

Guest Book: ✓ ✗

Entertainment: ....

Additional extras: ....

....

....

DJ/Band: ....

First dance: ....

Most vivid memory: ....

....

....

Funniest moment: ....

....

....

Most emotional moment: ....

....

....

What I may have done differently? ....

....

....

Wedding night was at:..

Favourite Gift received: ....

Other Details:..

....

....

Honeymoon: ....

*"Soulmates are people who bring out the best in you.
They are not perfect but are always perfect for you."*
AUTHOR UNKNOWN

 "Pachelbel Canon in D Major" (Johann Pachelbel)

YOU, ME AND OUR IDIOSYNCRASIES...

Every long-term relationship creates its own narrative, script, and routine, just between the two of you.

Your quirks, inside jokes & roles: ....

....

....

....

....

....

"Sometimes when you say 'Darling', I think you want to call me something else."

MARK JONES

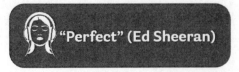 "Perfect" (Ed Sheeran)

IN LAWS AND OUT LAWS...

Relationships I have with my loved ones' loved ones:............................

....

....

....

....

....

....

"Men are what their mothers made them."
RALPH WALDO EMERSON

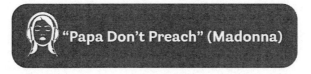

"Papa Don't Preach" (Madonna)

HEIR AND A SPARE...

Offspring:..

....

....

How we chose your name:..

....

....

....

Who you look like: ....

....

....

Character traits: ....

....

....

....

Significant events:..
....
....
....

I will always remember: ....
....
....
....

You can find a letter from me:...
....
....
....

"When I count my blessings, I count you twice."
BO LANIER

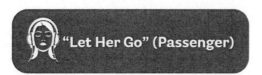
"Let Her Go" (Passenger)

OUR FAMILY...

Spouse/Partner Name:..

    D.O.B:...

    Nickname: ....

Children's Names (1): ....

    D.O.B:...

    Nicknames: ....

    Godparents: ....

    Grandparents:..

Children's Names (2): ....

    D.O.B:...

    Nicknames: ....

    Godparents: ....

    Grandparents:..

Children's Names (3): ....

    D.O.B: ....

    Nicknames: ....

    Godparents: ....

    Grandparents: ....

Children's Names (4): ....

    D.O.B: ....

    Nicknames: ....

    Godparents: ....

    Grandparents: ....

Children's Names (5): ....

    D.O.B: ....

    Nicknames: ....

    Godparents: ....

    Grandparents: ....

Stepchildren's Names (1): ....

    D.O.B: ....

    Nicknames: ....

Stepchildren's Names (2): ....

    D.O.B: ....

    Nicknames: ....

Stepchildren's Names (3): ....

    D.O.B: ....

    Nicknames: ....

Stepchildren's Names (4): ....

    D.O.B: ....

    Nicknames: ....

Siblings' Names (1): ....

    D.O.B: ....

    Nicknames: ....

Siblings' Names (2): ....

    D.O.B: ....

    Nicknames: ....

Siblings' Names (3): ....

    D.O.B: ....

    Nicknames: ....

Siblings' Names (4): ....

    D.O.B: ....

    Nicknames: ....

Nieces'/Nephews' Names (1): ....

    D.O.B: ....

    Nicknames: ....

Nieces'/Nephews' Names (2): ....

    D.O.B: ....

    Nicknames: ....

Nieces'/Nephews' Names (3): ....

    D.O.B: ....

    Nicknames: ....

Nieces'/Nephews' Names (4): ....

    D.O.B: ....

    Nicknames: ....

Nieces'/Nephews' Names (5): ....

    D.O.B: ....

    Nicknames: ....

Nieces'/Nephews' Names (6): ....

    D.O.B: ....

    Nicknames: ....

Godchildren's Names (1): ....

    D.O.B: ....

    Nicknames: ....

Godchildren's Names (2): ....

    D.O.B: ....

    Nicknames: ....

Godchildren's Names (3): ....

    D.O.B: ....

    Nicknames: ....

"Be yourself; everyone else is already taken."
AUTHOR UNKNOWN

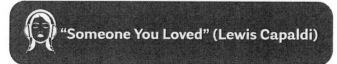 **"Someone You Loved" (Lewis Capaldi)**

SIBLING RELATIONSHIPS, ROLES AND RIVALRY...

....

....

....

....

....

....

"There are very few people in my life who have known every incarnation of me and have loved each one in turn, whilst also reminding me of the less lovable, numpty versions with pure, unadulterated delight! I love you, and I hope you love me."

LAURA BAKER

 "Wind Beneath My Wings" (Bette Midler)

WHAT'S MINE IS YOURS...

Important, sentimental Items:..

....

....

....

....

....

What I would like you to do with my possessions:...

....

....

....

....

....

The story behind them: ....

....

....

....

....

....

....

Please Keep: ....

....

....

....

....

....

....

Other:...

....

....

....

....

....

....

---

*"There are no goodbyes, wherever
you'll be, you'll be in my heart."*

GANDHI

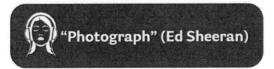

BEGINNING...

"Even the greatest was once a beginner.
Don't be afraid to take that first step."
MUHAMMAD ALI

 "The First Cut Is The Deepest" (Cat Stevens)

FIRST THINGS FIRST...

Talked: ....

Crawled: ....

Walked: ....

Cuddly Toy: ....

Memory: ....

House: ....

Nickname: ....

Pet: ....

Holiday: ....

Plane Journey: ....

Rode a Bike: ....

Best Friend: ....

Childhood Crush:..

Kiss:...

Date:..

Hobby: ....

School:...

Kids Club: ....

Award:...

Childhood Book: ....

Childhood Film: ....

Childhood Programme:...

School Performance:..

Embarrassing moment:...

Farcical 'fibs' my parents told me: ....

Fib to Parents:...

Loss: ....

Operation: ....

Puberty: ....

Job: ....

Wage: ....

How I spent my first paycheque: ....

Album: ....

Celebrity Crush: ....

Heartbreak: ....

Theatre/Musical Show: ....

Party: ....

Grown-up Kiss: ....

Date: ....

Piercing: ....

Alcoholic Drink: ....

Tattoo: ....

Driving Licence: ....

Vehicle: ....

Mates Holiday: ....

Festival: ....

Concert: ....

Home away from Home: ....

Other: ....

....

*"Enjoy the little things, for one day you may look
back and realise they were the big things."*
ROBERT BRAULT

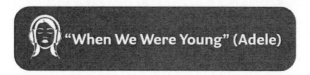
"When We Were Young" (Adele)

MY CHILDHOOD...

How & When My Parents Met: ....

Who I Lived With: ....

Family Pets: ....

My Parents' Jobs: ....

My Parents' Roles in the Household: ....

My Parents' Expectations of us: ....

Discipline: ....

Family Rules and Sayings: ....

Family Routines: ....

Regular Family Holidays: ....

Extended Family Relationships, relatives I regularly spent time with: ....

How we celebrated special occasions: ....

Happiest Times: ....

Hard Times that changed the family dynamics: ....

Three words that sum up my childhood: ....

Education: ....

Teenage Years:..

My Relationship with my Parents:..

What they taught me:..

What I would Change: ....

A Letter to my Younger Self:..

"Most of our childhood is stored not in photos, but in certain biscuits, lights of day, smells, textures of carpet."
ALAIN DE BOTTON

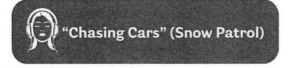
"Chasing Cars" (Snow Patrol)

HOW THE WORLD
HAS CHANGED...

I remember when...

A Loaf of Bread cost:..

Minimum wage was: ....

Phones were:...

A Freddo cost: ....

Average age to have children was:...

Most common names were:...

Dinner parties were normally:..

A can of pop was: ....

Popular slang words were: ....

Society 'frowned' upon: ....

Top Corporate names were: ....

Weddings were: ....

The Average House price was: ....

Top Fashion Brands were: ....

The legal age to drink was: ....

Popular Holidays were: ....

Big Charities were: ....

A Pint of Beer was: ....

Fuel cost: ....

Haircuts cost: ....

How the postal service operated: ....

Television was: ....

Language that was unacceptable: ....

Shopping was: ....

Passport Control was: ....

Pubs closed at: ....

It was illegal to: ....

Technology was: ....

You could leave education at: ....

You could get married at: ....

Other: ....

What I miss and the next generation will never experience: ....

Old Wives' Tales/Sayings: ....

New Inventions that shocked me: ....

"There is nothing permanent except change."
HERACLITUS

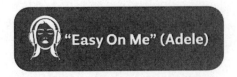
"Easy On Me" (Adele)

MY LOVED ONES WHO HAVE GONE ON AHEAD...

Who, when, how, favourite memories and what I will never forget.

Things that remind me of you.

What I loved most about you.

If I could have 5 more minutes with them.

....

....

....

....

....

....

....

....

....

....

....

....

....

....

....

....

....

....

....

*"If I could have 5 more minutes with you,
I would want 5 more minutes."*

JOLIE JONES

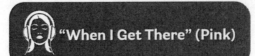 **"When I Get There" (Pink)**

FREESTYLE...

"Before you speak, let your words
pass through three gates:
Is it true?
Is it necessary?
Is it kind?"

BUDDHA

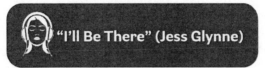